BANISHING BACKACHE AND DISC TROUBLES

An osteopath's searching investigation into the wide-spread complaint of backache and associated disorders, including disc troubles, with a penetrating analysis of causes and symptoms. Details of treatment are provided, based on sensible diet, corrective exercise, and relaxation. Backache — largely ignored by allopathic practitioners — can be banished by self-training, declares the author.

Banishing Backache and Disc Troubles

Harry Clements N.D., D.O.

THORSONS PUBLISHERS LIMITED
Wellingborough, Northamptonshire

First published 1952
Sixth Impression 1970
Second Edition, revised and reset, 1974
Second Impression 1975
Third Impression 1976
Fourth Impression 1979

ISBN 0 7225 0258 3 (paperback)
ISBN 0 7225 0358 X (hardback)

Typeset by Specialised Offset Services Ltd., Liverpool
and printed by Weatherby Woolnough
Wellingborough, Northamptonshire

Contents

Foreword

Very few people live their lives without experiencing backache in one form or another. It may be just a temporary inconvenience that comes and goes; quickly relieved, perhaps, with a little extra care and rest. On the other hand there are those for whom the problem is of far greater dimensions, occupying, as it were, a dominant place in the whole of their lives. The sufferer is never without his 'back', which interferes relentlessly with his work and his pleasures. It intrudes itself at all times during the daily tasks and may even interfere with rest and sleep.

In the past such sufferers appear to have received very little help from medicine, so that many of them regarded it as something that had to be patiently borne. While on every side their fellow-creatures might tell of the marvellous progress of medical science, no one seemed able to lift the burden of aches and pains that weighed upon their backs. They were relegated to the class of sufferers too ordinary to be noticed.

It may be said that since the advent of osteopathy there has been a brighter gleam of hope for these people, because it carried with it a new conception of the relationship between structure and function, and stressed the possibility that mechanical derangement could be a real causative factor, particularly in complaints like backache. From this standpoint body mechanics took on a new form and meaning; posture, balance and correlation became terms of great physiological significance, and were recognized as the bodily factors out of which most of the cases of intractable backache were created.

Out of this idea has grown a new conception of the inherent power of adjustability of the structure of the body, similar, indeed, to the inherent quality within us that heals our wounds, seals our cuts and reconstructs the broken bone. It is this concept that is important to the individual, because it emphasizes the importance of self-help both in the preventive and in the curative sense. The habits by which we have built up the structural pattern of our bodies (the bad ones of which have made manifest the ailments like backache and similar troubles) are modifiable by the exercise of will-power and self-training. It is with this point of view in mind that this book has been written.

I.
Backache: A Widespread Complaint

With perhaps the exception of headache, backache is the most common of all the symptoms of ill-health. There are very few people who have not suffered from it, and so little has been done in the ordinary way to meet this complaint that most people feel they have to put up with it. It may be because it is so common a symptom that so little has been done to meet it as a problem; there are many people who will say that they never mention the trouble to a doctor because they feel that medicine has so little to offer in the way of an effective remedy. It may be, they are wont to say, all right to take medicine for indigestion or constipation or some other such complaint, but there seems to be very little logic in taking it for a symptom like backache. In consequence, it becomes one of the commonest and one of the least regarded of all the burdens that the human has to bear.

Generally speaking, backache is regarded more as a nuisance than anything else, and very little sympathy is expended on its victims. It can be – and is – borne without too much outward manifestation, so that backache is usually suffered in silence, mostly on the assumption that it is a common trouble and a common lot.

DEFINITION OF BACKACHE

It is often very difficult to get the sufferer to give a clear definition of what is meant by this term. It seems to vary with almost every patient. One will complain that it is a sharp, painful symptom; another will refer to it as a dull ache; while another may describe it as a kind of weakness. It is often hard, therefore, to give it a definition that will apply to all the sufferers, and so we must content ourselves with a general one. Backache may be described as any aching pain affecting the structures of the body from the shoulders to the buttocks. Many people may think this too wide a region to be covered by the term, and usually confine it to a pain felt in the lower part of the back. But, as the pain is usually a radiating one, involving most of the large muscles of the back, it is wiser to think of it in a fairly wide sense.

MANY FORMS OF DISEASE

Backache is associated with various disease conditions, both acute and chronic. In acute diseases, like 'flu, and in the various infectious complaints, an aching back is almost an invariable accompaniment. Why this should be is not easy to explain, but some people do suffer very much in this way, and in rare cases the trouble may persist into what one may call an ordinary backache. Generally, however, with the passing of the acute illness the pain in the back clears also. This kind of a backache is, therefore, so far as we are concerned, not considered as a condition requiring special attention.

In some cases of so-called chronic disease there may be persistent backache. Many of the conditions that produce great debility lead to this symptom, and of course nothing save the successful treatment of the underlying disease will be of lasting value in clearing it up. The popular idea that backache is always associated with kidney trouble is not always true. It is true that in cases of established kidney disease there may be backache, but it is a fallacy to think that every backache indicates disturbance of the kidney and bladder functions, as some cleverly worded advertisements would have us believe.

Many internal troubles give rise to backache. Afflictions of the bowel, like colitis, for example, are almost invariably associated with this trouble, and the so-called fallen stomach also produces it. Pelvic disorders can cause it too, and haemorrhoids, or piles, may be an unsuspected cause. Without going into too much detail about these forms of backache, we want to make it quite clear that backache can exist, as it were, not within its own right, but merely as a manifestation of some disease condition. It should not, therefore, be overlooked merely as an isolated symptom.

LITTLE RELIEF FROM TAKING MEDICINE

Many sufferers are aware that very little relief is obtained from taking medicine. While this is never an advisable practice, there is no doubt that many other symptoms can be relieved in this way; but the weakness and persistence of backache seems to be not even temporarily amenable to these measures, and, as we shall explain later on, we believe that it is due to the fact that mechanical factors are involved. Now if proper measures are used in the alleviation of such mechanical factors no harm will accrue, no matter what the underlying condition may be; on the other hand, the taking of suppressive drugs may easily mask a situation that will go from bad to worse.

We desire to stress very strongly that the only way to give relief from backache safely is always to bear in mind that the structure of the body is under strain, and that whatever measure of relief is undertaken should be based on this premise. We should say to ourselves: what is it that disturbs the balance of the structure and thus produces the feeling of aching weariness of the back? We should remember at all times that we are dealing with a mechanical problem, and if we are able to solve the trouble along those lines we shall make a useful contribution to the health of the whole system.

A FERTILE FIELD FOR PHYSICAL TREATMENTS

The fact that medicine has been so ineffective in relieving backache has tended to make it a fertile field for what are known as physical treatments. Recently this has become increasingly widespread, and many facilities exist for this kind of treatment. Massage, heat and light treatments are often employed, and do indeed help to give some relief; but in many cases the point is overlooked that the underlying mechanical factor is not corrected. Such treatments may be given indefinitely, and tend to wear out the patient's confidence without solving the problem, so that after a time the course is abandoned.

The same applies to many forms of physical exercise. These are usually designed to strengthen the muscles, and the important factor of body balance is often left out of consideration. A person may have a well-developed physique and still suffer from backache and the disturbed body equilibrium that is usually associated with it. Even athletic training may not always produce the strong, supple, acheless back that one might imagine it would; and military training, although it has improved in recent years, has not always developed a back free from aches and pains. The point that is generally missed in these methods is that the body should be used with precision as a mechanical unit, with the balanced spine as both a flexible and supporting structure.

SYSTEMS OF SPINAL TREATMENT

There is no doubt that unrelieved backache has been one of the greatest problems of medical practice for many years, and it is very likely that out of this situation the various spinal systems developed. There is evidence that in primitive times the aching back was the concern of many people, and one of the most interesting methods of treating this condition was that of applying pressure to the spine. The patient would lie face down on the floor, and another person, sometimes a child, would walk up and down the spine, thus relieving the tension of the muscles. This method is, we understand, still practised in some primitive communities.

More recently bone-setters treated pains in the back by pressure and wrenching movements, and some of them became highly proficient in these methods. In the U.S. the very early osteopaths developed treatment along these lines, and made the discovery that the removal of aches and pains in the region of the spine appeared to have very beneficial effects upon other apparently unrelated illnesses. There can be little doubt that the persistent and unrelieved backache was the source from which these various practices started; and as the years have gone by, and more has been learned about the unity of the whole system, this manipulative technique has become of very great value.

THE ERECT POSITION OF THE BODY

A very important point that has been emphasized by the spinal therapists is the vital significance of proper bodily posture, in which the spine plays so large a part. The biped position, which gives the human so many advantages over the quadruped, is not without its disadvantages also. Maintaining erect position leaves the human open to a great deal of strain, and the constant struggle that he has to endure against the force of gravity may operate against him when his resistance is low. The quadruped, with his four supports, is at a much greater advantage than the biped so far as balance is concerned. And such equilibrium is a very complex mechanism for the two-legged creature. It keeps the anti-gravity muscles constantly on guard and the nervous system for ever maintaining it by reflex action. This struggle of the body for balance goes on from the time the child raises himself on his tiny feet until the aged and decrepit person finally gives it up.

A FLEXIBLE ROD

While all parts of the body are involved in the balancing mechanisms that sustain it in the erect position, the spine comes in for the major part of the work. The spine, as we all know, is a flexible rod, very cleverly contrived in its structures so that it gives strength for support and at the same time allows for free movements. For this reason it is formed into a series of well-developed curves, which ensures the greatest efficiency in this respect. The spine has to support the head, which is of considerable weight, and it is easy to understand that unless the head is easily balanced it throws a very great strain on the whole of the spine. About twenty different muscles are attached to the upper spine, and hence the free and easy movement of the head in relation to the rest of the body is very important. The middle of the spine, roughly speaking, is capable of very little movement because of the attachment of the ribs; but the lower part of the spine, the lumbar region, has to be capable of movement in varying directions, so that here we find a very powerful and flexible structure.

In the normal person the free and rhythmic play of the muscles of the body with every movement of the spine gives a very great measure of efficiency, which establishes the human body as a wonderfully effective instrument in both repose and action. But when this efficiency is disturbed, and especially when the flexibility of the spine is involved in the disturbance, the whole mechanical precision is impaired. That is just what happens when the back becomes the seat of aches and pains, and no one can mistake the burden it throws on its victim.

We should therefore always bear in mind that the erect position of the body and backache are usually very closely related. This will be a useful guide to us when we are looking for causes and planning helpful treatment.

RECOGNIZING MECHANICAL EFFICIENCY IN THE BODY

The old-fashioned idea that all the ills of the body could be cured by taking something into the stomach dies hard, and there are still many people who delude themselves with this notion. It is very difficult for them, if they still hold fast to this belief, to think in any other than chemical terms; and when a subject like backache is discussed they still want to believe that there must be some sovereign remedy — in a bottle. It has probably never crossed their minds that the body suffers aches and pains from structural and mechanical inefficiency, and they pay very little attention in their daily lives to the positions and habits they adopt which play so great a part in the making of troubles like backache.

For example, no person can really be physically efficient who may be suffering from some foot defect, even of a functional nature. A painful corn or an ill-fitting shoe will do more than just disturb the comfort of the foot; it will, unless it is quickly rectified, upset the whole equilibrium of the body. There is no doubt that flat or ill-functioning feet will have the same effect, and it is very difficult to estimate how many cases of backache have been due to the craze for high-heeled shoes.

STRUCTURAL CHANGES IN THE SPINE

It is easy to understand that when the natural position of the foot is grossly contorted, as it must be when very high heels are worn, some compensating changes must take place elsewhere in order to restore the balance. Such compensation usually takes place in the curves of the flexible spine, and if the condition persists over a long period structural changes may follow. The spine, as we have said, is a very flexible instrument, and in order that it should be so its structures must be very pliable and able to accommodate to practically any position; but if the position is retained over a long period certain changes may follow. For instance, the discs of the spine, those elastic pads between the spinal bones, change their shape with every movement; but if the spine becomes fixed at any point they may change their shape and lose their flexibility. Here you have the making of chronic backache, and the cause may seem unrelated to the back itself.

Anything, therefore, that interferes with the mechanical efficiency of the body as a whole is a potential cause of weakened structures in the back and, later, of the persistent chronic backache.

THE USE OF THE BODY

We are all brought up with the idea that the body will take care of itself, and we never regard it as an instrument that can be used or ill used by ourselves. It may have been true that when we lived in a more primitive way we were obliged to habituate ourselves to activities that called into play all the parts of the body, but under modern conditions it is quite common to over-use only one part. The difficulty that generally arises out of this is largely a postural one. We fall into the habit of sitting and standing badly; if this is not corrected by a conscious effort, postural strains will develop. The back, as we have already seen, will become the seat of many of them, and stage by stage the condition will deteriorate until the bad posture will interfere with the mechanical efficiency of the body.

The situation, then, calls for reconstruction of the bodily habits, so that the controlling mechanism, the nervous reflexes, will operate under favourable conditions. Put quite simply, it means that we have to look within ourselves for reform of the habits that are undermining the structural efficiency of the system. The first step will be to get the whole matter in better perspective — and that means we must do some thinking about it.

2.
The Causes of Backache

It is clear that backache, like so many other symptoms of an ill-functioning body, may be the result of many different causes. In this chapter we are discussing some of the most important ones, so that the reader will be able to analyse his own troubles in the light of these. We should always remember that there are causative factors at the back of all such symptoms, and if we are able to identify them it makes the task of planning effective treatment much easier. The art of finding basic causes is supposed to be the special province of the doctor, who is, of course, trained to make a diagnosis. But the patient, if he uses his own intelligence and observation, can often find them out for himself, and this will be of real assistance in overcoming the complaint.

FATIGUE AND STRAIN
People who suffer from backache nearly always suffer from fatigue also, and if we are able to find the cause of the fatigue the clearing up of the backache will not be difficult. Fatigue, one need scarcely say, is the result of strain. The strain may affect one both bodily and mentally, and its effect will be to lower the general resistance. Lowered resistance means that the

nervous system will not be able to carry out its function satisfactorily, and certain changes will wait upon this state of affairs. The waste products of the body, which should be quickly and properly eliminated, will be retained within the tissues, and, in Nature Cure terminology, there will be a toxaemic condition. The muscles and other supporting structures of the body lose their tone and efficiency, and chronic backache may develop.

Whenever we think about stress and strain, we must remember the vicious circle attendant upon them. If the strain is mental it may affect the physical also, and vice versa. If the strain is purely mechanical – such as, for example, straining the body by weight-bearing – it may affect the chemical side of the body by interfering with the elimination of poisons. If the strain is chemical – such as, for instance, constant indigestion – it may so disturb the general metabolism of the system that the muscles are weakened and unable to meet the normal stresses of life. Thus we see that strain may be one of the most important causes of backache, and there is no doubt that very few people are able to order their lives so as to avoid the strains that modern living constantly imposes.

But if we know just what the stresses are that we are bearing, then we may do much to counteract them and offset some of their more harmful effects. That is why we insist that searching for such strains is the most important thing to be done in the treatment of any kind of illness, and particularly one like backache. Unless we discover and remove the underlying causes we are only palliating the effects.

Some occupations give rise to straining positions of the body that may lead to backache. The same is true of various games. Without giving it much thought we slip into bad habits of standing, sitting and moving, and thus we may be using up much too much energy, besides putting certain structures of the body under undue strain. An adviser cannot follow a patient round watching how he deports himself at his work, in his games and his other activities, so the readjustment of such habits must be left to the discretion of the sufferer. A little thought turned inward on oneself, as it were, will in this respect be very well worth while.

RHEUMATISM AND FIBROSITIS

Of all the aches and pains that are felt in the region of the back, by far the majority are said to be due to either rheumatism or fibrositis. These terms are difficult to define, and they are generally used in a kind of blanket sense to cover almost any unusual sensation felt in the muscular structure. Basically speaking, fibrositis is used to denote a rheumatic affliction of the fibres of the muscles; but dividing up terms in this way is useful to no one.

In a recent discussion in a medical journal there seemed to be complete divergence of views between the various doctors. Some argued that the aches and pains in the muscles that were called fibrositis were nothing more or less than irritation of the spinal nerves, while others declared that the term fibrositis should be discarded because it was not really a definable condition. The whole discussion, it seemed, was productive of very little value, except that it showed that very few were able to agree on any given point of view.

In spite of this many people suffer from painful muscles in the back for which they seem to get very little relief from ordinary treatments. We think that these pains are more often than not related to, first, strain of the muscles and, second, fatigue and the retention within the tissues of the fatigue toxins. If we bear this in mind we shall be able not only to understand the cause that is operating but also to plan effective treatment.

MUSCLES LOADED WITH TOXINS

When a muscle is in a normal condition it contracts and relaxes smoothly and easily, thus controlling its circulation and disposing of its waste products. When not in action the normal muscle is soft and elastic, and causes no pain or unusual sensations. On the other hand, when a muscle is overstrained it loses the power of regulating its circulation, and the waste products of its activity remain within its fibre cells. The result is that the muscle is heavy and doughy and full of aches and pains.

Most so-called cases of fibrositis of the back are of this kind, and once this condition has developed the whole mobile efficiency of the back and the spine will be interrupted. When the muscles are loaded with toxins they are quite unable to respond to the normal impulses, and every movement leads to a great deal of discomfort. As we know, the muscles have to move the various joints in the spine; and every pull on them — and they are many in the course of ordinary activity — gives rise to some kind of pain. The result of this is that the pain tends to limit movement, and so the sufferer uses his muscles less and less. The fact that the muscles are not fully employed will in time tend to perpetuate the toxic condition, and so we have a vicious circle in operation.

This is the state of affairs that leads to muscular pains like lumbago in the lower part of the back. The same kind of pain may also be experienced in the middle and upper regions of the back, and is often described under different names. But the basic cause is very much the same, and the state of the muscular tissue will in all cases give a good indication of what the trouble really is. Such a condition is related to the general health, and all patients who are said to suffer from rheumatism and fibrositis of the back are in need of health-building measures.

Because of a lack of understanding of the basic cause of this condition many people do themselves much harm by self-medication. As a rule the medical man, because he is not very hopeful of helping the case, will not be over-enthusiastic about prescribing, and the patient, thrown back on his own resources, will look round for so-called household remedies. It is surprising how many people are willing to offer advice and suggest all kinds of remedies. Such remedies, although they can be easily obtained, are not always harmless. Used over long periods they do harm. The point is that this is no time for taking such things. As we shall show later, a proper course of health-building is needed to eradicate the trouble.

ARTHRITIS

A great deal of backache is caused by arthritis. Arthritis literally means inflammation of a joint, and was originally used because, no doubt, it was thought that the disease was confined to joints. We now know that although the joints are mainly affected, the complaint is in fact constitutional, and the inflamed and changing joints are the main symptoms. What concerns us here is that arthritis is the cause of much pain and discomfort in the back, both by virtue of the fact that it produces local changes in the many joints of the spine and the pelvis, and also because the changes that occur elsewhere in the body disturb the posture and thus cause backache.

Apart from the tissue changes that accompany it, arthritis always limits movement within a joint. The result is that the muscles and other structures associated with the joint no longer perform their normal function, so that in time changes take place in them also. When such a condition shows itself in the back it is bound to have far-reaching results. As we have already seen, mobility in the back is important at all times. So long as the spine is flexible, all the joints and the important discs are kept in normal condition. This constant movement keeps up the circulation, keeps the fibres elastic and maintains the pliability of the spinal curves.

SPINE BECOMES RIGID

As the arthritic condition develops it changes all this. The parts change and harden, and gradually the movement is lost. The curves are held rigid, and the discs, for want of normal use, lose their resiliency and shrink in size. The shock-absorbing qualities of the spine are lost, and it is only a matter of time before the whole spine becomes rigid. This is a state of affairs from which the spinal structures will not easily recover.

Arthritis usually starts at one point in the spine and then gradually involves the other parts. Apart from the actual progressive nature of the disease, there is no doubt that in the early stages many mistakes are made in handling the complaint so that other parts are often made susceptible. For instance, the patient may, in order to relieve the pain or for some reason, carry his body in such a position as to throw undue strain on the other regions of the back. Now nothing will make any joint in the body susceptible to this trouble like strain. It lowers the resistance and allows the waste products to be retained. Thus the part becomes a fertile spot for the arthritic toxins which are already developing within the system.

In addition, therefore, to basic methods to eradicate the disease, great care should be taken to see that the effects of joint involvement do not throw further strain upon other parts, and very much can be done in this way in helping the body to compensate for such changes and strains. As a general rule one need not be afraid of movement in an arthritic joint; a patient is very unlikely of his own accord to do any damage by keeping up the normal function of a joint, which is, of course, active movement.

COMPENSATING CHANGES

The development of arthritis in other parts of the body may lead directly to backache. When this disease starts in the lower limbs and affects the joints of the feet, knees and hips, it is more than likely that much pain and discomfort will be felt in the back, because it is here that so many compensating changes will have to be made. The whole balance of the body will have been undermined, and the weight-bearing mechanisms will be badly strained. Often this throws a strain through the pelvic joints, the sacro-iliac, and when this great shock-absorbing area has been disturbed the whole spine above it will be in a precarious condition. The arthritic joint in the lower members may alter the level of the pelvic bones, so that there will be a one-sided pull on the big lumbar muscles. When these great guy ropes of the spine are placed at such a disadvantage anything may happen to the structures of the back. The natural adjustability of the tissues will be lost, and a sudden fall or wrench will mean a definite injury to the affected parts.

Arthritic joints in the feet may readily cause aches and pains in the back. These troubles may make a start in one foot and thus cause an uneven distribution of the body weight. This will inevitably throw strain on other compensating joints, and, in the way already explained, the arthritic toxins may soon find another region lessened in resistance and ripe for their development.

AILMENTS OF THE DIGESTIVE TRACT

In many cases of stomach and bowel disorders backache is a common symptom. When these cases are of an acute nature all of the symptoms, including the backache, will soon disappear. But this should show us the relationship between chronic digestive and bowel disorders and persistent backache. This has not been sufficiently realized, and because of this oversight many intractable cases of backache have failed to respond to treatment.

At present it is probably very difficult to find a person with a normal digestive tract. There are so many factors abroad to upset it. Apart from constant strain of modern living there is the danger of food sophistication in which so many agents are employed to change the nature of food. These agents must have some effect on the digestive system, but not even the best-informed chemists are fully aware of what these effects may be. These agents certainly interfere in some measure with normal digestion and thus cause a strain on the system. Such digestive irritation will set up reflex actions in the spinal nerves and tissues, and if the condition is allowed to continue, very painful symptoms will develop in the muscles of the upper part of the back. Many people who have suffered in this way have been treated for fibrositis or some other form of rheumatism when the seat of the trouble lay in the stomach itself.

Another condition that may lead to the same symptoms is the constant distension of the stomach. People who suffer from dyspepsia find that their stomachs appear to be 'blown out', and in fact they are by the delayed digestive processes. As a result the large abdominal muscles, which should act in unison with the movements of the ribs, become immobile, and in consequence the chest walls are limited in movement. This limitation of movement is later transferred to the spine and the back muscles, and the symptoms show themselves as pains in the back and round the ribs.

CONSTIPATION CAUSES BACKACHE

Constipation or disorder of the bowels has been blamed for a good many different complaints, from headache to cancer. Whatever truth there may be in such contentions, it is certainly a common cause of backache. This is often overlooked, and many different kinds of treatment for backache fail because they do not rectify this underlying cause. Those who practise spinal therapeutics are aware that sluggishness of the bowels gives rise to all kinds of painful spots in the tissues of the back, and they know also that when the bowel is restored to its normal condition these irritating areas will clear up. A great many aches and pains in the back are often attributed to other factors, and the real seat of the trouble, the bowel, is often unsuspected.

HARMFUL TREATMENTS

Unfortunately much of the treatment used for the correction of bowel disorders is more harmful than the complaint itself. The idea has grown up that the evacuation of the bowel is synonymous with normality, so that if the bowel 'moves' then the whole matter has been rectified. From this standpoint many people argue that if they take some kind of remedy to 'move' the bowel all will be well. This idea is totally false, and a great deal of harm has resulted from it. It has been responsible for the laxative and purgative habit, which is probably one of the most pernicious of all forms of medication.

When this habit is carried on — as it is by a great many people — as a daily performance, the bowel tends to become exhausted, and the constant irritation, especially of the lower bowel, leads to a certain amount of congestion. The accompanying and irritating piles are resultant upon this congestion, and a persistent backache will almost certainly follow. In classifying laxatives as herbal or vegetable or otherwise it is important to remember that if they cause an exaggerated action of the colon their continual use will lead to chronic constipation. In short, there is no known way of overcoming constipation except by regarding it as a symptom of a disorder that involves not only the parts affected but the whole personality, and then by readjusting the health-destroying habits that have made it possible.

It should be remembered that when digestive and bowel disorders persist over a period there will be a definite tendency for the organs and tissues of the abdomen. There will not be much hope of overcoming the resulting backache until the sagging organs have been restored.

WOMEN'S TROUBLES
Most women in the course of life suffer from backache in one form or another. Difficulties with the menstrual period are generally held to be largely responsible, and some women are inclined to regard

the trouble as a part of their common lot. This is quite the wrong attitude to adopt, because there is reason to think that all such natural functions should be without pain. A careful analysis of such cases will often show that other accompanying complaints, such as constipation, are more definite contributing factors. By improving the general health and restoring the tone of the muscular system, which often means paying strict attention to diet and to a sensible course of exercise, the sufferer may look forward to complete relief.

Many women suffer from backache after confinement, especially if it has been difficult. Here we have to think in terms of strain and its after-effects. During confinement a great deal of strain is thrown upon the large sacro-iliac joints and the various structures related to them, and this may remain the cause of a lot of back trouble. Nowadays more attention is paid to proper preparation for confinement by the practise of exercises and relaxation, but there are still many women who do not recover their normal body balance after childbirth and suffer much backache in consequence.

In many such cases the actual painful symptoms do not develop for some time after the confinement, and there may be a tendency then to overlook the strain of the confinement as a causative factor and to label the complaint as fibrositis. The massage and light treatment which is so often employed for fibrositis will not make much impression on sacro-iliac strain, and unless the whole outlook is changed the ground will have been prepared for chronic backache. In trying to assess the causes of backache a mother should always look back to the possibility of a confinement as a starting point, and especially if she was subjected to prolonged strain at that time.

POSTURE AND BACKACHE

In a sense poor posture and backache are almost synonymous terms; the conditions that promote the one promote the other also. For example, the strain of childbirth, which strains the sacro-iliac joint, will cause backache, and poor posture will always be associated with it. Indeed, practically all the causes so far mentioned produce their harmful effects on the back by way of their deteriorating effects on the bodily posture.

Thus in effective treatment for backache we must always attend to the posture of the body. There is no exception to this; but it must be remembered that the removal of the basic cause does not always restore proper posture. For instance, backache caused by sluggishness of the bowels is rectified by attention to diet, and the improvement in the bowel action will give some, but perhaps not complete, relief to the backache. This is because at the time when the bowel was functioning badly the spine was strained and some of its flexibility was lost. For complete restoration it will be necessary to reassess the body balance and by suitable measures make sure that it has been returned to normal.

3.
Symptoms of Backache

It is easy to say that a pain in the back covers most of the subject, but a closer examination will show that the symptoms are often varied and associated with many bodily disorders. It is very rare indeed to find a patient with just a simple localized pain in one part of the back; more often than not it ties up with many other disturbances.

One of the most common symptoms associated with backache is nervous tension. The patient feels tense and irritated, and if this is allowed to persist he will complain of nervous exhaustion. The fatigue will interfere with both physical and mental activities, and the patient will become aware of a feeling of ineffectiveness. The backache will seem to be in the background of these nervous complaints, and the individual will feel that if that could be overcome all the other symptoms would vanish also. The fact that no relief seems to be forthcoming adds to his depression.

Backache of some kind is almost always associated with the so-called neurasthenic state. In these cases the sufferer appears to pay more attention to his nervous symptoms than to his backache, but he will admit its presence in any analysis of his general symptoms. What he has probably forgotten is that the backache preceded his other symptoms, and this is often significant for future treatment.

DIFFICULTIES OVERLOOKED

Many people treat their symptoms as they turn up. If there is a pain in the throat, then the throat is treated; if there is headache, something is taken to relieve it; and so on. The real danger in this is that the more fundamental difficulties are overlooked, and conditions like backache will persist to set up remote manifestations.

In this respect we might cite cases of neuritis. The pains of this disorder, which are felt in the arms, chest, legs and other parts, are practically always secondary to neglected backache, and many patients are deceived because of this. They suppose that the parts of the body where they feel the pain should receive the treatment, and they often waste much time and effort in applying various external applications. This is typically true of sciatica, where the seat of the trouble is in the lower part of the back but where very little pain is experienced as a rule. Neuritic conditions often bring with them difficulties of the circulation, and it is very common to find swollen hands and feet that are closely related to backache that has existed over a long period.

HEADACHE AND NECK MUSCLES

Another often unsuspected ailment closely related to back troubles is a certain form of headache that causes much distress and is unresponsive to ordinary treatment. The seat of the trouble is in the strained condition of the neck muscles, and the various nerves in that area are irritated, leading to painful symptoms throughout the scalp area. The headache may be very persistent, and the muscles of the scalp will be very sensitive to the pressure of the fingers. Brushing the hair and even washing the head will seem to add to the irritation. This condition always goes with a badly balanced spine and the nervous tension that accompanies it.

There are many internal conditions that may suggest the thought that actual disease exists, whereas in fact the symptoms are reflex conditions related to the backache. Pains in the intercostal muscles (between the ribs) may be thought to be due to pleurisy, whereas the real seat of the trouble is in the irritated spinal nerves. Pains in the chest, which are sometimes thought to be related to the heart or lungs, are of a similar nature. Many cases of pain in the muscles of the abdomen, near the appendix region, have been diagnosed as appendicitis but eliminated by treatment that restored the integrity of the spinal nerves. Osteopaths have been accused of trying to cure appendicitis by manipulation because they have cleared up such conditions wrongly diagnosed by others.

The main point to bear in mind about these various aches and pains is that if there is at the back of them, as it were, a long-standing backache, this should be considered as a possible source of the trouble. In any case the removal of the backache is of paramount importance and should not be looked on as something that may be suffered without causing disturbances elsewhere.

EFFECTS OF DIFFERING POSITIONS OF THE BODY

In some cases of backache the symptoms are not manifested until the body assumes certain positions. Some people can adopt a standing position without much discomfort, but when they sit or lie down the back begins to ache. Conversely, the symptoms are brought on in the standing position. These symptoms often relate to the usage of the body in various occupations. A man, for example, may work all day at the bench and his back may appear to be easily adjusted to the various positions that he has to adopt. If he has to assume one special position like, say, standing sideways and using his two hands as a carpenter might use a plane, it may be found that his back seems to be under no strain whatsoever. But when he sits or lies down painful spots may develop in the spinal muscles. This will probably be because his position at work tends to overstrain one group of muscles and leave another undeveloped.

Such a form of backache may unsuspectedly undermine the general health. If, as usually happens, it comes on after a short period of sleep, it will tend to rob the sufferer of his normal rest and his general bodily resistance will be placed under strain. Such cases often go untreated because the patient is unable to relate the trouble to any apparent cause, and in consequence may not seek advice. If he seeks advice at all, he is more likely to seek it for sleeplessness, and the usual insomnia remedies will deaden the discomfort and leave him tired and depressed when morning comes.

It may therefore be taken as a general rule that there is some strain and tension in the spine if it is not possible to assume all ordinary positions without feelings of pain and discomfort. The best way to meet these difficulties is to undergo a course of self-training to restore the balance of the whole spine, and to develop an awareness of right and wrong usage of the body during ordinary occupations. The longer these strains and tensions are 'put up with', the more difficult the task will be of overcoming them. A mechanical strain of this nature does not get well of its own accord; indeed, it almost always tends to deteriorate.

LUMBAGO AND SCIATICA

In days gone by the term lumbago was applied to almost all painful conditions of the lower part of the back. More recently the term 'low back pain' came into use, and now many people use the term 'slipped disc'. As a matter of fact the old idea about lumbago was a fairly good one, because it described an acute condition closely related to a so-called chill or cold; and today many sufferers do not get the proper treatment because they think that the trouble is due to an injury and thus neglect the need for constitutional treatment.

We should use the term lumbago, if we use it at all, to denote a condition where there is an excruciatingly painful condition of the big lumbar muscles which is usually associated with a cold or some slight elevation of the body temperature. Such a condition usually attacks those who suffer from backache in the ordinary way, and these acute attacks show that restorative treatment is needed between attacks to take the strain of the lumbar muscles and rid them of their fatigue poisons. These fatigue toxins are probably at the bottom of the acute attacks, because they make the muscles susceptible to chills and colds. As a rule the attack increases the circulation through the muscles and clears up, for the time being, the retained waste products. Therefore soon after the acute attack has subsided, treatment should be started to restore the balance of the whole spine and to strengthen the muscles.

The symptoms of lumbago need very little description. A back that is painful in almost any resting position and agonizing in movement covers the matter. The cough, which sometimes accompanies it when the patient has a cold, will seem to break the back, just as sneezing will also. These very acute attacks generally subside quickly, but they may leave behind a painful and somewhat intractable condition: sciatica. This means that the congested and inflamed condition of the back muscles has probably spread to the sheath of the great sciatic nerve trunk — the largest in the body — and from then onward the leg affected may be the seat of an intense aching pain. Again, it is not necessary to describe these symptoms in any detail. They are familiar to most people. Suffice it to say that it is one of the most painful of complaints, which reduces the patient's efficiency in many ways and robs him of most of the joys of living.

TENDERNESS IN THE PELVIC JOINTS

Another symptom associated with backache is tenderness in the pelvic joints. As most people know, the spine is superimposed upon a wedge-shaped bone, the sacrum, that fits, keystone-like, between the two great pelvic bones, and the junctions of these bones are called the sacro-iliac joints. These joints can be felt under the fingers as heavy ridges, and it is here that tender spots show themselves. Sometimes the patient can feel them on movement, but generally they do not bother him very much except when they come under pressure. Sometimes, also, one can feel under the fingers little movable lumps, called nodules, which are very painful when pressed.

These conditions show that the pelvic joints are under postural strain, and they give rise to many unsuspected symptoms in other parts of the body. These joints are essentially shock-absorbers, and under strain they lose this important function. The result is that the shocks are transferred to the spine and are conducive to headaches. No person can have normal lightness of step and carriage if the sacro-iliac joints are under strain, and the general health will greatly improve when the joints are normalized.

BACKACHE IN CHILDREN

The symptoms of backache are sometimes overlooked in young children. Children are rarely asked if they are conscious of such a weakness, yet many suffer in this way. Many children, when they complain of pains in the limbs and back, are told that they are suffering from 'growing pains', and they then regard them as a part of the growing period of their lives. Such a term should never be used because there is no such condition, and pain of any kind is related to abnormal function and never to normal function. Such pains indicate that there is some disorder that needs attention, and in many cases they relate to postural strain.

4.
Disc Troubles and Backache

Until about the early 1930s very little attention was paid to the spinal disc, and certainly before this time it was rarely mentioned in articles and books dealing with backache and sciatica. Anatomists knew, of course, that it played an important part in the functioning of the spinal column, but apparently no one regarded it as a possible cause of pain and discomfort. When it was learned that changes could take place in the disc that would cause troubles, it became almost a new fashion in everyday complaints. These changes were due mainly to protrusion of the disc, which might have been due to a prolapsed condition or to its having herniated or burst. The misplaced part of the cartilage caused pressure on the nearby nerves and thus set up intense pains, which were felt not only in the back but in the legs as well, because the great sciatic nerve was involved. This condition could arise in any part of the spine but was most likely to occur in the lower part of the back and in the upper region of the spine, and from the latter it might cause neuritis in the shoulders and arms.

'SLIPPED DISC'
As such cases have been more frequently seen and

diagnosed, a new term has crept into use. Anything appearing to resemble this condition is spoken of as a 'slipped disc', and no work on backache would be complete it if did not pay some attention to it.

A few words must be said about the structure and function of the spinal disc so that the reader will understand the problems involved. The spine is essentially a flexible rod made up of bones, ligaments and other structures, and formed into definite curves. Its main function is to protect the vital spinal cord, but it also has to provide support and at the same time allow for the various movements of the body. In order to give this resiliency to the structure the soft, yielding discs are placed between the bones, and thus a ball and socket joint is formed which is only limited in movement by the other structures.

The disc is therefore an elastic pad shaped to fit between the surfaces of the bones. The outer part of the pad is made of strong tough fibres, arranged criss-cross, to add to the strength, while the inside of the pad is formed of a soft compressible material. When all the structures are normal this inner material not only moves with each movement of the spine, but acts as a shock-absorber to the many jars and shocks to which the spine is constantly subjected.

One has only to think for a moment to realize just how important this part of the spine must be in everyday activities. When one is standing for long periods, a great deal of strain is placed directly on it, and that is why at the end of the day we may find the body height slightly diminished. These pads have been compressed. Think how much depends on these pads when you are running and jumping and the constant shock-like effects are being driven through the spine. Unless the discs are functioning properly the effects of the shocks will be felt in the head, and the whole nervous system may be upset. When we are young these pads are soft and pliable, and so we are able to run and jump about with very little concern to ourselves; when we are old and the pads have lost their elasticity such activities are difficult and even dangerous. When people suffer from disease such as arthritis these pads may be affected, and are no longer able to absorb shocks or allow free movement of the spinal joints.

SOME MISTAKEN NOTIONS ABOUT THE PROBLEM

Many people have a completely erroneous notion about what has happened when they develop disc trouble. The term 'slipped disc' gives them the impression that one of the discs has slipped bodily out of place. When we see how strongly the spine is bound together we realize how impossible this is. An injury violent enough to do this would probably spend itself in fracturing the bones of the spine.

What has actually happened in most cases is that the pad has either burst and its inner part protruded, or a section of it has given way. The injury is serious because the protruding part can cause pressure on the nerve trunks which lie in the vicinity and thus set up painful reactions elsewhere. The difficulty of repairing the damage must be apparent to everyone; first of all, cartilage does not mend easily; secondly, the parts involved are under constant strain; and thirdly, immobility of the parts may undermine the integrity of the whole spine.

These cases of actual breakdown of the discs are much rarer than is generally imagined. Not every stab in the back means a damaged disc, and not every doctor's diagnosis of such a condition is right. It is very difficult to be absolutely sure about such a diagnosis; indeed, only the surgeon who opens the spine can be certain of the condition, because the ordinary X-ray may miss it completely.

CAUSATIVE FACTORS IN DISC TROUBLES

In almost every case of such disc troubles the spine must have experienced some kind of violence. Such violence need not have been spectacular. A listing job of some kind, or a false step, may have been sufficient to provide the last straw – and usually it is a question of the last straw. A healthy and flexible spine can withstand an enormous amount of shock and strain before anything gives way.

The integrity of the spinal structures may be undermined in many ways. Inadequate nutrition may be one of them. This does not mean that under-feeding is a cause, nor that the lack of red meat is the only factor in under-nutrition. The trouble is more likely to be the over-eating of deficient foodstuffs like white flour and white sugar and the foods made from them. Such foods lack the important mineral salts, and this may be a contributing source of the complaint.

Anything that weakens the spinal discs will tend towards the final breakdown. The various positions of the body, if maintained over too long a period, may strain a spinal disc. For example, sitting for long periods may tend to round out the back and at a certain point compress one or more of the discs. Continued over the years, this may leave a very weak spot that only requires a sudden jerk to cause a protrusion of the discs.

The breakdown often occurs when one has a cold and all the muscles of the body are inclined to ache. Sedentary workers especially should avoid any strain-ing movement when they suffer from a cold or even the first signs of one; the idea of 'working it off' is one of the most dangerous things anyone may do.

THE SYMPTOMS OF DISC TROUBLES

The general idea is that there are no warning symptoms for this complaint — that it occurs suddenly and without relationship to any other factor. This is by no means always true. A careful analysis of cases will show that weakness in the back has been a common symptom and has too often been disregarded. The truth is that the suddenness and painfulness of the last attack is so great that it obliterates memory of other things.

The chief symptom, then, is the sudden and excruciating pain, the 'stab in the back'. Quickly following this is the rigidity of the muscles of the lower back. Often this rigidity applies more to one side than the other, and thus the body is slung to one side, just as though the spine were badly curved. Walking is performed with great effort, and every movement of the legs brings intense pain.

After the acute pain in the back has subsided, the effect of the pressure on the nerves will be felt in the leg, and then we say that the patient is suffering from sciatica. The pains may vary in different parts of the body, depending on the nerves that are involved. As we have already said, the discs of the lower or upper spine are the ones usually affected, and so the pains are felt mostly in the legs and in the arms. Generally, the symptoms of the condition known as 'slipped disc' are related to the sciatic nerve, and sciatica is the main symptom.

TREATMENT: SOME ESSENTIAL POINTS

The general treatment plan we shall discuss in our next chapter will apply equally to 'slipped disc' cases, but a few points are of special interest to these sufferers. The first is that it is vitally important, in the very early stages of the attack, to lose no time in planning effective treatment. Taking aspirin or some other pain-killer, and trying to carry on, is a great mistake which will lead to further complications. As soon as the attack occurs, therefore, a period of absolute rest is needed. This should be continued until the muscles of the back have lost their rigidity.

The resting position is very important. It should be on a bed that is firm, and the best position of the body is face downwards. This is because it is important to restore the curves in the lower back. As we know, the normal curve in the lower spine is well forward, but it will be found that when disc trouble exists the spine will either be almost completely straight or even tend to curve backwards. By lying on the face the spine is allowed to fall forward, as it were, and thus the big lumbar muscles will be able to relax or 'let go'.

In this position it is useful to apply hot fomentations to the lower back to reduce the pain and rigidity of the muscles. If the sufferer is troubled with sluggishness of the bowels, and they are overloaded, a warm-water enema will give more relief than purging medicine. In all such conditions the healing, self-repairing power of the body is helped either by staying on a very light diet or, better still, by living entirely on liquids such as fruit juices and vegetable juices. It is important at such times to increase the intake of water, which should be taken as water and not as an addition to tea, coffee and the like.

When the acute stage has passed and the patient returns to more or less normal activity, a certain amount of careful self-training will be necessary. The main point to remember is that the inward curve of the lower spine must be maintained. This should be carefully observed when standing and sitting. Occasionally place the hands on the lower spine when in the standing and the sitting positions, and try to adjust the rest of the body so that the lower back is forced inwards. Afterwards learn to assume a position that tends to maintain this inward curve.

5.
Treatment (1)

The first thought to have in mind in the treatment of backache, or for that matter any other such symptom, is the general health of the whole body. We should never think of any part of the body as an isolated structure that bears little relationship to the body as a complete unit. All the parts are linked one to the other by the blood, the nerves and the intercommunicating tissues. In this sense we may rightly use the analogy of the machine, in which the absence of one part or the wrong adjustment of another may upset the whole equilibrium.

We use the term 'general health' to signify a condition in which all the functions are being carried out properly and smoothly. The process of digestion, the process of elimination and the mechanism of respiration are among the many functions that must be working efficiently to maintain the balance of general health, and we cannot hope to cure or eliminate a symptom like backache unless we carry this concept in our minds.

ATTACKING SPECIFIC WEAKNESSES THAT MAY EXIST

It is clear that with a trouble like backache certain

weaknesses may exist within the system which should receive special treatment. These are generally due to mechanical factors that impose undue strains on the spine. Most of these cases will need very careful reorganization of all the daily habits of living, because the real causative factors lie chiefly in habits built up in the course of our lifetime.

Our daily habits chiefly relate to food and the care we take of the digestive and eliminative systems, plus the mechanical usage of our bodies during our many activities. Generally speaking, every case of backache should be considered from these two important aspects. Very few such cases will not respond to the following commonsense methods.

THE QUESTION OF DIET

Many people still think that diet applies only to diseases like diabetes, where there is direct evidence that food is an important factor. From the Nature Cure viewpoint diet is important in every condition both of health and of ill-health, not only because it supplies the body with essential materials, but because its proper regulation may be an important factor in the natural healing processes of the system. This concept is based on an entirely different one from that which underlies the practice of medicine. In Nature Cure terminology we regard all disease processes as related to what we term toxaemia. We use this term not, as is ordinarily done in medicine, to signify actual blood poisoning, but as indicative of a condition of the blood, the lymph and the cells where the normal waste products of the system have been retained beyond the normal period.

When the body is functioning normally – that is, when it is in a state of health – the intake and output of the assimilative and eliminative processes are in a state of equilibrium. On one side of this balance we have the digestive system, and on the other the great depurating organs, the bowels, the kidneys, the skin and the lungs. The digestive system breaks down and dissolves the food we take into the alimentary tract and passes it into the lymph and the blood for use by the cells of the tissues. It is in the cells that the vital assimilation takes place. Now the cells are little systems in themselves, which not only need nutriment but constantly develop waste products from their own activity. The nutrients and waste products are transported through the blood and the lymph, and the efficiency of the whole system depends on the relationship between the digestive system, the blood and the lymph and finally the cells which form the tissues and structure of the body.

When this relationship is upset we get a breakdown of the various functions. We may get digestive and bowel disorders because the system is no longer able to make full use of the normal amount of food, and on the other hand we get a slowing up of all the eliminative processes with the resultant retention within the blood and lymph and tissues of the waste products of vital activity. In this state of bodily affairs, which is at the basis of all disease conditions, we are faced with the fact that the intake of food, even if the food is of normal quality, may add to the stress and strain of the system and probably do more harm than good.

From this point of view food may play a tremendous part in restoring the efficiency of the body. We do not imply by this that food contains within itself some curative principle, as so many people mistakenly think, but rather that the regulation of the food itself, in quality and quantity, will enable the system to regain its normal digestive and assimilative balances.

THE VALUE OF FASTING

In chronic complaints like backache it would be impossible to find a case that did not show all the symptoms accompanying this initial toxaemia, and as a first step in practical dietetics the withholding of food for a short period is of inestimable value in restoring the normal equilibrium.

Let the sufferer think this matter over for himself, and he will be convinced that giving the whole system a rest in this manner is only a matter of common sense. Let him think for how long he has taken his three or four meals a day irrespective of the needs and the capacity of his body, and he will soon appreciate how much he has contributed to his own undoing through constantly disturbing and over-straining the digestive-assimilative processes. Let him not say that it does not apply in his case; it applies in every case of ill-health. In every case like backache that has persisted over a fairly long period we can be fairly certain that there will be congested muscular areas where the fatigue and other toxins are retained. So many of the cases that are termed fibrositis are cases of this nature, and no treatment is of much avail until these toxins have been released. Withholding food takes the load off the great transport system of the body, the blood and the lymph, and clears up these congested areas as no other method will.

It might therefore be laid down as a rule that in all cases of backache the first step in treatment should be a short period of abstinence from food. Such a period may be from one to three days' duration, and it is better to have it at weekly or bi-weekly intervals rather than to undertake a long fast. Such a short period will not interfere with one's normal activities, or at any rate it will barely take up more time than a weekend. If the backache is related to other disturbances of the system this should not necessarily prevent one from undertaking this period of digestive rest. Half the common ailments from which so many people suffer would disappear if the digestive organs were rested in this way.

Backache arising mainly from over-distension of the stomach and bowels will be quickly relieved by this simple procedure, and the reduction in the body girth that will ensue will make the patient feel as if a weight has been taken off his back. Relieving the system in this way will add to the mobility of the abdominal muscles, which will be followed by easier and fuller breathing, which again may clear up long-standing pains in the upper back and shoulders.

PLANNING A SENSIBLE NORMAL DIET

The planning of a sensible diet is very easy if we are willing to be guided by a few simple rules. The chief difficulty is that all the dietitians and scientists have been so busy making researches into the constituents of food that the ordinary person sheers off because he thinks the whole subject is so complicated. Take, for example, the case of vitamins. So many have been discovered, and so much has been done about them in relation to various disease conditions, that this part of dietetics alone entails almost a lifetime study. The same is true of mineral salts, or, for that matter, the protein, fat and other constituents of food. The ordinary person may therefore argue that he does not know just where to begin or where to leave off.

But people should remember that in trying to separate all these various parts of our foods we are only separating that which nature has organized in her great laboratories, and that, indeed, we are not able to reconstitute them even in the state of our present scientific knowledge. To make this point quite clear let us think of wheat. This cereal is practically a complete food as it is organized by nature. We have not, however, been satisfied to use it in that form, so we have divided it up into various foodstuffs and vitamin preparations. The part we use as flour for breadmaking is generally about 70 or 80 per cent extraction, and the remainder may be divided up into many other forms. The bran may be used for the treatment of constipation because it contains roughage and certain other substances. The germ of the wheat is rich in vitamins and is used as a food supplement. The oil is rich in vitamin E, and is therefore used for its effects upon fertility; and so on. Thus to use wheat in the way we commonly do we must have extensive knowledge of the puzzle we have made for ourselves, and have skill in order to apply such knowledge in a practical way.

The point is that whilst no one wishes to discourage those who want to pursue these studies, there is no need for anyone to forget the simple truth that food is always better balanced, so far as the individual's nutrition is concerned, by being used in its natural state – i.e., as nearly as possible in the condition in which nature has organized it. In the present order of our society we admit that we cannot follow this rule entirely, but we still can do a great deal about it. We can apply it to many foods in daily use – fruits, vegetables, cereals and so on; and if we do, it will solve most of the vitamin and mineral salts problems that appear to be so confusing.

THE IMPORTANCE OF PROPER FOOD COMBINATIONS

Some years ago Dr Tilden worked out a plan for

combining foods that has since met with a great deal of misrepresentation. In spite of this it is a very useful and practical plan, and is to be highly recommended, especially to those who want to work out their own diet. The chief feature of the plan was the separation of foods rich in protein from those rich in starch. For instance, Dr Tilden argued that it was wrong to follow a meat course with a heavy starchy pudding. For those whose digestions were already disordered he went so far as to say that starchy foods like potatoes should not be eaten with meat, fish, etc., and made the same prescription with starch and eggs and cheese. His opponents came back with the argument that there was nothing in psysiology to justify such a rule and that nature had combined starch and protein in many foods, as for example in beans and in many other vegetables. But reducing the idea to this point missed the whole force of Dr Tilden's argument.

Dr Tilden was not really concerned with digestion and the physiological effects of food at all; he was concerned with stress and its effects upon the individual. For instance, if the individual eats a heavy meal it places a strain upon the whole system, and it scarcely matters what kind of foods are eaten. On the other hand, a light meal lessens such a strain. Now meals that contain both protein and starch are more likely to be difficult of digestion. The conventional meal of soup, meat and pudding is a good example.

The importance of Dr Tilden's plan is that it is the most practical yet devised for the arrangement of the normal diet. During the course of the day the body should be supplied with all the food elements, and we can arrange the three meals to meet this requirement without throwing any strain on the digestive system. This is of the greatest importance to anyone who